Managing Diabetes with Diet

Mastering Low GI & High Protein Meals

by Bruce Goldwell

Disclaimer:

The information provided in this book is intended for general informational purposes only and is not a substitute for professional medical advice, diagnosis, or treatment. Always seek the advice of your physician or another qualified health provider with any questions you may have regarding a medical condition. Never disregard professional medical advice or delay in seeking it because of something you have read in this book.

The author and publisher of this book are not responsible for any specific health or allergy needs that may require medical supervision and are not liable for any damages or negative consequences from any treatment, action, application, or preparation, to any person reading or following the information in this book.

Every effort has been made to present accurate and up-to-date information at the time of publication. However, the author and publisher do not make any representation or warranties with respect to the accuracy, applicability, fitness, or completeness of the contents of this book. They disclaim any warranties (expressed or implied), merchant-ability, or fitness for any particular purpose.

The use of any information provided in this book is solely at your own risk. The author and publisher shall have no liability or responsibility to any person or entity regarding any loss or damage incurred, or alleged to have been incurred, directly or indirectly, by the information contained in this book. It is recommended that readers verify any information obtained from this book and consult with a qualified healthcare professional for specific health concerns.

The inclusion of specific products or brands in this book does not imply endorsement or recommendation. Product information is provided for informational purposes and should not be considered as an endorsement of any particular product.

By reading this book, you acknowledge and agree to these terms and conditions.

Table of Contents

Managing Diabetes with Diet

"Wisdom isn't knowing everything-

it's knowing when to learn from others."

Introduction

This comprehensive guide has been meticulously structured to walk readers through every essential aspect of incorporating a low glycemic index (GI) and high protein diet into their daily lives, aiming for a profound and positive impact on health and well-being. From the foundational understanding of the glycemic index and its significant health implications to the practical applications that bring this knowledge to life through a diverse array of recipes, the guide is crafted to ensure a seamless educational journey.

Building Blocks to Mastery:

The journey begins with the basics of the glycemic index, offering readers a solid grounding in what GI is, how it's measured, and why it matters to our health. This foundational knowledge is crucial as it sets the stage for understanding the broader implications of dietary choices on blood sugar levels, weight management, diabetes control, and overall metabolic health.

Progressive Learning Approach:

As the guide progresses, it builds on the initial concepts introduced, layering in the complexities and nuances of choosing low GI, high protein foods. This methodical approach ensures that readers are not just passively consuming information but are actively engaging with the material, making connections between dietary choices and their direct effects on health and wellness.

Practical Applications and Recipes:

Recognizing that knowledge is most powerful when put into practice, the guide transitions from theory to action, providing readers with practical tools and a wide range of recipes. This section is designed not only to inspire but also to demonstrate how low GI, high protein foods can be deliciously incorporated into daily meals. The recipes serve as a direct application of the concepts discussed, offering tangible ways to make healthier food choices without sacrificing flavor or satisfaction.

Repetition for Retention:

Within the guide, certain core principles and information may be reiterated across different sections. This intentional repetition is a pedagogical strategy designed to reinforce key concepts, ensuring that readers fully absorb and understand the information presented. By encountering these principles in various contexts—from theoretical explanations to practical cooking tips—readers are more likely to internalize the lessons and apply them to their own lives.

Comprehensive Understanding for Lifestyle Integration:

The ultimate goal of this structured approach is to equip readers with a comprehensive understanding of low GI, high protein diets, empowering them to make informed dietary choices that enhance their health and well-being. By the guide's conclusion, readers should feel confident in their ability to integrate these nutritional principles into their daily routines, making choices that support stable blood sugar levels, optimal health, and a vibrant lifestyle.

In summary, this guide is more than just a collection of dietary advice and recipes; it is a roadmap to a healthier way of living. By carefully building on foundational knowledge, reinforcing key concepts through repetition, and providing practical applications, it aims to transform readers' approach to food and nutrition, paving the way for lasting health benefits.

Preface

The Importance of Understanding the Glycemic Index

In our journey towards optimal health and wellness, understanding the foods we eat and their impact on our bodies is crucial. The Glycemic Index (GI) stands out as a pivotal tool in this quest, offering insights into how different foods can influence our blood sugar levels. Developed in the early 1980s by Dr. David Jenkins and his colleagues, the GI has transformed the way we view carbohydrates, providing a scientific basis for making healthier food choices.

The GI ranks foods on a scale from 0 to 100 based on how they affect blood sugar levels compared to pure glucose, which has a GI of 100. This ranking system divides foods into three categories: low GI (55 or less), medium GI (56 to 69), and high GI

(70 or more). Understanding these categories and the GI values of foods empowers us to make choices that can stabilize blood sugar levels, which is especially beneficial for weight management, diabetes control, and overall health.

Why is this important? Fluctuations in blood sugar are not just a concern for those with diabetes. They affect our energy levels, mood, hunger, and even long-term health, including risks for heart disease and obesity. By choosing foods with a low GI, we can maintain steadier blood sugar levels, leading to improved energy, satiety, and a reduced risk of chronic disease.

Moreover, the GI concept has evolved to include the Glycemic Load (GL), a more nuanced measure that considers the carbohydrate content in a serving size of food, offering a fuller picture of a food's impact on blood sugar. Together, GI and GL are invaluable tools for anyone looking to adopt a healthier lifestyle.

This book aims to demystify the glycemic index and its implications for your diet. By understanding and utilizing the GI, you can make informed decisions that contribute to a balanced, nutritious diet, supporting both your immediate well-being and long-term health. Whether you're looking to manage your weight, control diabetes, maintain healthy blood pressure, or simply eat better, the insights and recipes provided here will guide you on your journey to a healthier life.

Join me as we explore the significance of the glycemic index, the benefits of low GI diets, and how to incorporate high-protein, low GI foods into your meals. With this knowledge, you'll be equipped to create a diet that not only tastes good but also brings you closer to your health goals.

The Evolution of the Glycemic Index

A Brief History

The story of the Glycemic Index (GI) begins in the early 1980s, marking a significant milestone in nutritional science. Its development is credited to Dr. David Jenkins, a professor at the University of Toronto, who, along with his colleagues, sought a method to classify carbohydrates based on their immediate impact on blood glucose levels. This pioneering work led to the introduction of the GI, a tool that has since revolutionized dietary planning and management, particularly for individuals with diabetes.

Before the advent of the GI, carbohydrates were generally considered as a single group, with little differentiation regarding their effects on blood sugar. The prevailing thought was simple: all carbs raised blood glucose levels, and managing intake was a matter of controlling quantities. However,

Dr. Jenkins' research introduced a nuanced perspective, revealing that not all carbohydrates affect blood sugar in the same manner. This insight was groundbreaking, showing that the type of carbohydrate mattered just as much as the amount.

The initial study that gave rise to the GI involved feeding carbohydrate-rich foods to healthy volunteers and measuring their blood sugar responses. These responses were then compared to the effects of pure glucose, which has the highest GI value of 100. Foods that led to a slow, gradual increase in blood sugar were ranked lower on the index, while those causing a rapid spike were ranked higher. This differentiation allowed for a more sophisticated approach to dietary management, especially important for those needing to monitor their blood glucose levels closely, like people with diabetes.

The introduction of the GI sparked a paradigm

shift in nutritional science and dietetics. It underscored the importance of the quality of carbohydrates in managing health and disease prevention. Subsequent research expanded on Jenkins' work, exploring the implications of low-GI diets for weight management, cardiovascular health, and metabolic syndrome, among other conditions.

The GI's evolution did not stop with its initial development. The concept of Glycemic Load (GL) was later introduced to provide an even more accurate assessment of a food's impact on blood sugar. GL takes into account both the GI of a food and the amount of carbohydrate it contains per serving, offering a more comprehensive picture of how a food might influence blood glucose levels over time.

Today, the Glycemic Index is a cornerstone of contemporary nutritional advice, influencing dietary recommendations worldwide. Its development has empowered millions to make more informed food choices, leading to better blood sugar control and improved overall health. The GI continues to be a subject of research, with scientists exploring its applications in various dietary contexts and its potential for addressing global health challenges.

As we delve deeper into the benefits of low-GI diets and explore high-protein, low-GI recipes, it's important to appreciate the historical context and scientific innovation that gave us this valuable dietary tool. The Glycemic Index remains a testament to the ongoing quest for knowledge in the service of human health, offering a path to more personalized and effective nutritional strategies.

Understanding the Glycemic Index

What is the Glycemic Index?

Definition and Development

The Glycemic Index (GI) is a scientific ranking that classifies foods based on their impact on blood glucose (sugar) levels. It provides a numeric scale ranging from 0 to 100, where pure glucose, a simple sugar that serves as a reference point, is assigned a GI of 100. Foods are measured against this standard to determine how quickly they raise blood sugar levels after consumption. The GI is an essential tool for anyone looking to manage their blood sugar, whether for weight control, diabetes management, or overall health.

The development of the GI was a groundbreaking moment in nutritional science, introduced by Dr. David Jenkins and his team at the University of Toronto in the early 1980s. The team's research aimed to address a crucial gap in understanding how different carbohydrate-containing foods affect blood sugar levels. Before the GI, carbohydrates were broadly categorized as either simple or complex, based on their chemical structure. However, this classification did not accurately reflect how these foods influenced blood sugar levels upon digestion.

Dr. Jenkins' work involved feeding volunteers various carbohydrate-rich foods and then measuring their blood glucose responses over time. These responses were compared to the effects of consuming an equivalent carbohydrate amount from pure glucose. The results of this research led to the establishment of the GI scale, where foods that cause a rapid and high increase in blood sugar are rated closer to 100, and those that result in a slower and lower rise are rated closer to 0.

The GI categorizes foods into three main groups:

- Low GI (55 or less): These foods are digested and absorbed slowly, resulting in a gradual rise in blood sugar and insulin levels. Examples include most fruits and vegetables, legumes, and whole grains.
- Medium GI (56 to 69): Foods in this category cause a moderate increase in blood sugar. Examples include some rice varieties, rye bread, and sweet potatoes.
- High GI (70 or higher): These foods lead to a rapid spike in blood sugar and are typically processed or refined carbohydrates, such as white bread, most white rices, and sugary cereals.

Understanding and utilizing the GI can significantly impact dietary planning, especially for individuals with metabolic conditions like diabetes. By choosing lower GI foods, one can achieve better blood sugar control, which is crucial for managing diabetes and reducing the risk of developing type 2 diabetes in at-risk individuals. Furthermore, incorporating low GI foods into one's diet supports weight management strategies by promoting longer periods of satiety and reducing the likelihood of overeating.

The GI's development has not only enhanced our understanding of carbohydrates and their effects on the body but also provided a practical tool for making healthier food choices. By selecting foods with a lower GI, individuals can support their health goals, from improving blood sugar management to achieving and maintaining a healthy weight.

Understanding GI Values and Their Significance

Understanding the Glycemic Index (GI) values of foods and their significance is crucial for anyone looking to manage their diet for health, weight loss, or blood sugar control. The GI scale, which ranges from 0 to 100, categorizes foods based on how quickly and significantly they raise blood glucose levels after being consumed. This section delves into the nuances of GI values and why they matter for your health and dietary choices.

GI Values Explained:

- Low GI Foods (55 or lower): These foods are absorbed and digested slowly, leading to a gradual increase in blood sugar and insulin levels. Incorporating low GI foods into your diet can help manage hunger and maintain energy levels throughout the day, making them especially beneficial for weight management and blood sugar control. Examples include legumes, whole grains, nuts, seeds, and most fruits and vegetables.

- Medium GI Foods (56 to 69): Medium GI foods cause a moderate rise in blood sugar levels. They can be included in a balanced diet but should be balanced with low GI foods to moderate blood sugar spikes. Examples include some varieties of rice, pasta, and some bread.

- High GI Foods (70 or higher): High GI foods result in rapid spikes in blood sugar and insulin levels. Regular consumption of high GI foods can lead to energy crashes and may increase the risk of developing type 2 diabetes and cardiovascular diseases. These include white bread, white rice, and sugary snacks.

The Significance of GI Values:

1. Blood Sugar Management: For individuals with diabetes or pre-diabetes, understanding GI values is essential for maintaining blood sugar levels

within a healthy range. Choosing lower GI foods can prevent the sharp spikes in blood sugar that contribute to the long-term complications associated with these conditions.

2. Weight Control: Low GI diets promote satiety and reduce hunger, which can help with weight management. By favoring slow-releasing energy foods, you're less likely to experience the rapid hunger that comes after consuming high GI foods, potentially reducing overall calorie intake.

3. Energy Levels: Foods with lower GI values provide a more consistent energy supply, whereas high GI foods can lead to energy peaks followed by crashes. For sustained energy throughout the day, incorporating low GI foods into meals and snacks is beneficial.

4. Reduced Disease Risk: Studies suggest that diets high in low GI foods are associated with a

reduced risk of developing type 2 diabetes, heart disease, and certain types of cancer. The slow and steady blood sugar response elicited by low GI foods may contribute to this protective effect.

5. Nutritional Quality: Often, low GI foods are also high in fiber, vitamins, and minerals. Choosing these foods contributes to overall nutritional well-being and supports long-term health.

Understanding and applying GI values in daily eating habits can have profound effects on health and well-being. It's not just about choosing foods with the lowest GI but about balancing your diet to include a variety of nutrients while managing blood sugar levels. For those looking to optimize their health, understanding the GI and incorporating its principles into dietary choices is a powerful strategy.

Glycemic Index vs. Glycemic Load

The Difference Explained

While the Glycemic Index (GI) provides valuable insights into how different foods affect blood sugar levels, the concept of Glycemic Load (GL) extends this understanding by taking into account the quantity of carbohydrates in a serving of food. Together, GI and GL offer a more comprehensive approach to managing dietary choices for better health outcomes.

Glycemic Index (GI): As previously discussed, the GI ranks foods on a scale from 0 to 100 based on their impact on blood sugar levels compared to pure glucose. It is a measure of the quality or speed of carbohydrate digestion and subsequent effects on blood sugar levels.

Glycemic Load (GL): GL, on the other hand, combines the GI value with the actual carbohydrate content in a portion of food to give a more accurate picture of a food's real-life impact on blood sugar. It is calculated by multiplying the GI of a food by the number of carbohydrates in grams provided by a serving of that food and dividing by 100. The result is a number that classifies the food's impact on blood sugar based on both the quality and quantity of carbohydrate it contains. GL values are categorized as low (10 or less), medium (11 to 19), and high (20 or more).

The Importance of Both in Dietary Choices

Understanding both GI and GL is crucial for making informed dietary choices, particularly for individuals managing diabetes, looking to control weight, or simply aiming to maintain stable energy levels throughout the day. Here's why both metrics are important:

Comprehensive Blood Sugar Management: While GI provides a basic understanding of how quickly a carbohydrate is converted into glucose, GL offers a more complete picture by considering how much carbohydrate is in a serving of food. This distinction is vital because a food with a high GI may not significantly impact blood sugar levels if only a small amount of carbohydrate is present.

Informed Dietary Planning: Knowing the GI and GL of foods can help individuals plan meals that stabilize blood sugar levels. For example, pairing a high GI food with foods that have lower GI and GL values can balance the meal's overall impact on blood sugar.

Weight Management and Health: Diets with a focus on low GI and GL foods are associated with reduced risk of developing type 2 diabetes, cardiovascular disease, and certain cancers. They also promote satiety, which can aid in weight management by reducing the likelihood of overeating.

Enhanced Nutritional Quality: Foods with low GI and GL values tend to be richer in fiber, vitamins, and minerals. Incorporating these foods into one's diet supports overall health and well-being.

Understanding the nuances between GI and GL empowers individuals to make dietary choices that can lead to more stable blood sugar levels, better health outcomes, and improved quality of life. By considering both the quality and quantity of carbohydrates in foods, individuals can tailor their diets to meet their specific health goals, ensuring a balanced and nutritious approach to eating.

The Benefits of Low Glycemic Diets

Weight Loss and Low Glycemic Diets

How Low GI Aids in Sustainable Weight Loss

Low glycemic (GI) diets have become increasingly popular in weight management strategies, not just for their immediate impact on blood sugar levels but for their long-term benefits in sustainable weight loss. Understanding how low GI foods contribute to weight loss can help individuals make informed choices about their diets, leading to healthier lifestyles and successful weight management.

Stabilizing Blood Sugar Levels: Low GI diets are centered around foods that cause a slow, gradual rise in blood sugar and insulin levels. This stability is crucial for weight loss because it helps prevent the spikes and crashes that can lead to increased hunger and overeating. By maintaining steadier blood sugar levels, low GI diets can reduce cravings and help control appetite, making it easier to stick to a healthy eating plan.

Increasing Satiety: Foods with a low glycemic index tend to be more satisfying than their high GI counterparts. They take longer to digest and absorb, which means they stay in your stomach longer and help you feel full for an extended period. This increased satiety can lead to a natural reduction in calorie intake, as individuals may find themselves eating less frequently or consuming smaller portions.

Improving Fat Oxidation: Some research suggests that low GI diets may enhance the body's ability to burn fat as fuel, instead of storing it. This improved fat oxidation can contribute to weight loss and is particularly beneficial for those looking to not only lose weight but also improve their body composition by reducing body fat percentage.

Supporting Metabolic Health: Low GI diets have been linked to improvements in various metabolic health markers, including reduced insulin resistance and lower levels of blood lipids. These changes can support weight loss efforts and reduce the risk of developing metabolic syndrome and type 2 diabetes, conditions often associated with obesity.

Encouraging Healthy Eating Patterns: Finally, low GI diets naturally encourage the consumption of whole, unprocessed foods such as fruits, vegetables, legumes, and whole grains. These foods are not only low in GI but also rich in nutrients and dietary fiber, which are essential for overall health and can help with weight management.

Incorporating low GI foods into your diet is a practical and effective strategy for achieving and maintaining a healthy weight. By focusing on the quality of carbohydrates and choosing foods that promote satiety and metabolic health, individuals can enjoy a variety of nutritious foods while working towards their weight loss goals. Sustainable weight management is about making informed dietary choices that support long-term health and well-being, and low GI diets offer a scientifically backed approach to achieving these objectives.

Managing Diabetes with Low GI Foods

The Role of Low GI in Blood Sugar Control

For individuals living with diabetes, managing blood sugar levels is a crucial aspect of maintaining overall health and preventing complications associated with the condition. Incorporating low glycemic index (GI) foods into the diet is a strategic approach that can significantly aid in blood sugar control. This section explores the role of low GI foods in diabetes management and how they contribute to stabilizing blood glucose levels.

Improved Glycemic Control: Low GI foods are digested and absorbed more slowly than high GI foods, leading to a gradual rise in blood sugar levels rather than sharp spikes. For people with diabetes, this slow release is beneficial as it helps manage postprandial (after eating) blood glucose and reduces the risk of hyperglycemia (high blood sugar). Consistent consumption of low GI foods can improve glycemic control, a critical factor in managing diabetes effectively.

Enhanced Insulin Sensitivity: Regular intake of low GI foods can also improve insulin sensitivity over time. Insulin sensitivity refers to how effectively the body uses insulin to lower blood glucose levels. Improved insulin sensitivity means that the body requires less insulin to control blood sugar levels, which is particularly beneficial for individuals with type 2 diabetes, who often experience insulin resistance as a central feature of the disease.

Reduced Risk of Hypoglycemia: For those on insulin or certain diabetes medications, maintaining stable blood glucose levels is essential to avoid hypoglycemia (low blood sugar), a potentially dangerous condition. Low GI foods provide a more consistent energy release, which can help prevent the sudden drops in blood sugar that lead to hypoglycemia, making them a safer choice for diabetes management.

Supporting Weight Management: Obesity and overweight are significant risk factors for the development of type 2 diabetes. Low GI diets not only help in blood sugar control but also aid in weight management by promoting satiety and reducing overall calorie intake. Since weight loss can improve insulin sensitivity and glycemic outcomes, incorporating low GI foods into a diet plan can be a dual-purpose strategy for individuals with diabetes.

Long-Term Health Benefits: Beyond immediate blood sugar control, a low GI diet can have broader health benefits for people with diabetes. Studies suggest that such diets can improve cholesterol levels, reduce inflammation, and lower the risk of heart disease, which people with diabetes are at increased risk for. Thus, managing diabetes with low GI foods aligns with a holistic approach to health, addressing both glucose regulation and the prevention of diabetes-related complications.

Incorporating low GI foods into a diabetes management plan requires understanding the GI values of foods and learning how to balance meals for optimal glycemic control. By choosing low GI carbohydrates and combining them with healthy proteins and fats, individuals with diabetes can enjoy a diverse, nutritious diet that supports blood sugar stability, enhances overall health, and improves quality of life.

Low GI Diets and Blood Pressure

The Connection Between Low GI Foods and Heart Health

Low glycemic index (GI) diets are not only beneficial for blood sugar management and weight control but also have a significant impact on blood pressure and overall heart health. The relationship between low GI foods, blood pressure regulation, and cardiovascular wellness is complex and involves various physiological mechanisms. Understanding this connection can empower individuals to make dietary choices that support heart health alongside other health goals.

Promoting Vascular Health: Low GI diets contribute to improved vascular function by facilitating better blood sugar control and reducing insulin resistance. High insulin levels and blood sugar fluctuations can impair blood vessel function and increase the risk of hypertension (high blood pressure). By stabilizing blood sugar levels, low GI foods help maintain healthy blood vessels, which is essential for normal blood pressure regulation.

Reducing Inflammation: Chronic inflammation is a known risk factor for the development of hypertension and cardiovascular diseases. Low GI diets, rich in whole grains, legumes, fruits, and vegetables, are associated with lower levels of inflammatory markers. These diets are high in antioxidants and phytonutrients, which combat inflammation and protect against vascular damage, thereby supporting heart health.

Aiding Weight Management: Obesity and overweight are significant risk factors for hypertension. Low GI diets support sustainable weight loss and weight management by enhancing satiety and preventing overeating. By facilitating weight control, low GI diets indirectly contribute to lower blood pressure and reduced strain on the heart.

Improving Lipid Profiles: Diets consisting of low GI foods have been shown to improve lipid profiles by reducing levels of LDL (bad) cholesterol and increasing HDL (good) cholesterol. Improved lipid profiles are crucial for heart health, as high levels of LDL cholesterol can lead to atherosclerosis (plaque buildup in the arteries), increasing the risk of high blood pressure and coronary heart disease.

Encouraging Healthy Dietary Patterns: Low GI diets naturally encourage the consumption of a variety of nutrient-dense, minimally processed foods. This dietary pattern is aligned with broader dietary recommendations for cardiovascular health, such as the DASH (Dietary Approaches to Stop Hypertension) diet and the Mediterranean diet, which emphasize fruits, vegetables, whole grains, and healthy fats.

Supporting Long-Term Cardiovascular Health: The benefits of low GI diets extend beyond immediate blood pressure regulation. By contributing to weight management, reducing inflammation, improving lipid profiles, and promoting overall healthy dietary patterns, low GI diets play a significant role in the prevention of long-term cardiovascular conditions, including heart disease and stroke.

In conclusion, the connection between low GI foods and heart health is supported by evidence linking these dietary choices to improved blood pressure control, vascular function, and overall cardiovascular wellness. Adopting a low GI diet can be a key component of a heart-healthy lifestyle, offering a proactive approach to reducing the risk of hypertension and related cardiovascular conditions.

A Healthy Heart and Low Glycemic Diets

Preventing Cardiovascular Disease through Diet

The link between diet and heart health is well-established, with low glycemic (GI) diets emerging as a powerful tool in the prevention of cardiovascular disease (CVD). By focusing on the quality of carbohydrates consumed, individuals can significantly impact their risk factors for heart disease, emphasizing the role of diet in maintaining cardiovascular health. This section explores how low GI diets contribute to heart health and the prevention of cardiovascular disease.

Stabilizing Blood Sugar Levels: Chronic high blood sugar and insulin resistance are significant risk factors for the development of cardiovascular disease. Low GI diets help stabilize blood sugar levels and improve insulin sensitivity, reducing the stress on the cardiovascular system. By mitigating these risk factors, low GI diets play a critical role in heart disease prevention.

Lowering Inflammation: Inflammation is a key contributor to the development of atherosclerosis, a condition characterized by the buildup of plaque in the arteries, leading to heart disease and stroke. Diets rich in low GI foods are associated with reduced levels of inflammatory markers. This anti-inflammatory effect is partly due to the high fiber, antioxidant, and phytonutrient content of many low GI foods, such as fruits, vegetables, and whole grains.

Improving Blood Lipid Profiles: Low GI diets have been shown to positively affect blood lipid levels, including reducing total cholesterol and LDL (bad) cholesterol while increasing HDL (good) cholesterol. These changes in lipid profiles decrease the risk of plaque buildup in the arteries, directly contributing to heart health and reducing the risk of coronary artery disease.

Aiding in Weight Management: Obesity and overweight are significant risk factors for cardiovascular disease. Low GI diets support weight loss and management by promoting satiety and helping control appetite, which can lead to a reduced caloric intake and healthier body weight. Maintaining a healthy weight is crucial for reducing the burden on the heart and preventing hypertension, a major risk factor for CVD.

Promoting Healthy Blood Pressure: Hypertension, or high blood pressure, is a leading cause of heart disease. Low GI diets, by virtue of their emphasis on whole, nutrient-dense foods, can help maintain healthy blood pressure levels. This effect is enhanced by the inclusion of potassium-rich foods, common in low GI diets, which support vascular health and blood pressure regulation.

Encouraging Overall Healthy Eating Patterns: Adopting a low GI diet encourages a pattern of eating that aligns with other heart-healthy dietary approaches, such as the Mediterranean and DASH diets. These eating patterns are rich in fruits, vegetables, lean proteins, and healthy fats, all of which contribute to cardiovascular health by reducing disease risk factors.

Incorporating a low GI diet as part of a comprehensive lifestyle approach to health can significantly reduce the risk of developing cardiovascular diseases. By focusing on the quality of carbohydrates and prioritizing whole, nutrient-rich foods, individuals can positively impact their heart health. Prevention through diet offers a proactive means to combat one of the leading causes of morbidity and mortality worldwide, demonstrating the power of nutrition in maintaining a healthy heart and reducing the prevalence of cardiovascular disease.

Foods and Food Groups

Exploring Low GI Food Groups

Comprehensive Guide to Low GI Foods

Understanding and incorporating low glycemic index (GI) foods into your diet is a key strategy for maintaining stable blood sugar levels, supporting weight management, and reducing the risk of chronic diseases. Low GI foods are digested and absorbed at a slower rate, providing a gradual release of sugar into the bloodstream. This section offers a comprehensive guide to food groups rich in low GI options, helping you make informed choices for a balanced and nutritious diet.

Whole Grains: Whole grains are an excellent source of low GI carbohydrates. Unlike refined grains, they retain the bran and germ, providing fiber, vitamins, and minerals. Examples include:
- Barley
- Bulgur

- Quinoa

- Rolled or Steel-Cut Oats

- Whole Grain Pasta

Legumes: Legumes are not only low in GI but also high in protein and fiber, making them an excellent choice for blood sugar control and heart health. Some of the best options include:
- Black Beans
- Chickpeas
- Lentils
- Kidney Beans
- Soybeans

Fruits: While the GI of fruits can vary, many are low to medium on the GI scale and can be included in a low GI diet. They are also rich in fiber, vitamins, and antioxidants. Low GI fruits include:
- Apples
- Berries (strawberries, blueberries, raspberries)

- Cherries

- Grapefruit

- Oranges

- Pears

- Plums

Vegetables: Most non-starchy vegetables have a low GI and are packed with nutrients. They can be consumed in generous amounts for their health benefits. Low GI vegetables include:
- Broccoli

- Carrots

- Cauliflower

- Leafy Greens (spinach, kale)

- Peppers

- Tomatoes

Dairy and Dairy Alternatives: Dairy products and their alternatives can be part of a low GI diet. They provide calcium, protein, and other essential nutrients. Look for:

- Milk (especially low-fat or non-fat)

- Yogurt (plain, with no added sugar)

- Soy Milk

- Almond Milk (unsweetened)

Nuts and Seeds: Nuts and seeds are low in GI and offer healthy fats, protein, and fiber. They are great for snacks or as additions to meals. Include options like:
- Almonds

- Chia Seeds

- Flaxseeds

- Peanuts

- Walnuts

Meats and Fish: While not a source of carbohydrates, lean meats and fish complement a low GI diet by providing high-quality protein and essential fatty acids without affecting blood sugar levels. Opt for:
- Chicken or Turkey Breast (skinless)

- Lean Beef or Pork

- Fatty Fish (salmon, mackerel, sardines) for omega-3 fatty acids

Incorporating a variety of foods from these low GI food groups can help ensure a balanced diet rich in essential nutrients while managing blood sugar levels effectively. When planning meals, consider the overall balance of macronutrients (carbohydrates, proteins, and fats) and aim to include at least one low GI food in each meal or snack. This approach not only aids in glycemic control but also supports overall health and well-being.

Navigating High GI Foods

Foods to Limit and How to Balance Them

While incorporating low glycemic index (GI) foods into your diet is beneficial for maintaining stable blood sugar levels and overall health, understanding how to navigate high GI foods is equally important. These foods can cause rapid spikes in blood glucose, which can be particularly concerning for individuals with diabetes, insulin resistance, or those looking to manage their weight. This section provides guidance on high GI foods to limit and strategies for balancing them within your diet.

High GI Foods to Limit:

1. Refined Grains and Their Products: White bread, white rice, and foods made from refined flour like pastries and some crackers have a high GI and are low in fiber. These should be consumed

sparingly.

2. Sugary Snacks and Beverages: Candy, cookies, sodas, and other sugary drinks quickly elevate blood sugar levels and offer little nutritional value. They are best limited in any healthy diet.

3. Processed Foods: Many processed foods, including fast foods, are not only high in GI but also in unhealthy fats and additives. Opting for whole, minimally processed foods is a healthier choice.

4. Some Starchy Vegetables and Fruits: Potatoes, pumpkin, and watermelon have higher GI values compared to other vegetables and fruits. While still nutritious, they should be balanced with lower GI foods.

Strategies for Balancing High GI Foods:

1. Combine with Low GI Foods: When consuming a high GI food, pair it with low GI foods to help moderate the overall impact on your blood sugar. For example, add vegetables to a pasta dish or have a salad with your pizza.

2. Incorporate Protein and Healthy Fats: Including a source of protein or healthy fats with a high GI meal can slow the absorption of sugar into the bloodstream. Adding chicken to a rice dish or avocado to a slice of toast can help.

3. Watch Portion Sizes: Being mindful of portion sizes is crucial. You can enjoy high GI foods occasionally, but keep portions small to minimize their impact on your blood sugar.

4. Focus on Whole Foods: Even when choosing higher GI foods, opt for those that are less

processed. Whole grain bread, for example, may have a moderate to high GI but is a better choice than white bread due to its additional nutrients and fiber.

5. Physical Activity: Engaging in physical activity, especially after consuming a high GI meal, can help lower blood sugar levels. A walk or light exercise post-meal can be beneficial.

6. Balance Throughout the Day: If you consume a high GI food in one meal, aim for lower GI choices in your other meals or snacks throughout the day to maintain balanced blood sugar levels.

Understanding how to navigate high GI foods is not about strict avoidance but about making informed choices that support your health goals. By applying these strategies, you can enjoy a varied diet that includes occasional high GI foods while still managing your overall glycemic load effectively. This balanced approach promotes not only blood sugar control but also a sustainable, enjoyable eating pattern.

High Protein, Low GI Foods

The Importance of Protein in a Low GI Diet

Integrating high protein, low glycemic index (GI) foods into your diet is a strategy that offers multiple health benefits, enhancing not only blood sugar stability but also supporting weight management, muscle health, and overall satiety. This combination is particularly powerful for individuals looking to improve their metabolic health, manage or prevent diabetes, and sustain a healthy lifestyle. Here's an exploration of the benefits of high protein, low GI foods and their importance in a balanced diet.

Optimized Blood Sugar Control: One of the primary advantages of consuming high protein, low GI foods is the improved regulation of blood sugar levels. Protein has a minimal impact on blood glucose levels and can help moderate the effects of carbohydrate consumption by slowing digestion and the absorption of sugar into the bloodstream. This results in a more stable and gradual rise in blood sugar levels, which is crucial for preventing the spikes and crashes that can lead to insulin resistance and diabetes over time.

Enhanced Satiety and Weight Management: High protein foods are known for their ability to promote feelings of fullness, which can help reduce overall calorie intake by decreasing hunger and the desire to snack between meals. When combined with the slow-release energy from low GI carbohydrates, this effect is amplified, making it easier to manage weight and prevent overeating. This is particularly beneficial for individuals looking to lose weight or maintain a healthy weight without feeling deprived.

Support for Muscle Health and Recovery: Protein is essential for the growth, repair, and maintenance of muscle tissue. Incorporating high protein, low

GI foods into your diet ensures that your muscles receive the nutrients they need, especially after exercise. This is important for everyone, from athletes to those engaged in regular physical activity, as it supports muscle recovery and helps maintain lean muscle mass, which is key for a healthy metabolism.

Increased Nutritional Value: High protein, low GI foods often come packed with essential nutrients, including vitamins, minerals, and dietary fiber, contributing to overall health and well-being. Foods such as legumes, lean meats, dairy products, and certain whole grains provide a rich source of these nutrients while adhering to the principles of a low GI diet.

Diverse Dietary Options: Emphasizing high protein, low GI foods in your diet doesn't mean sacrificing variety or flavor. There is a wide range of foods that fit these criteria, offering ample opportunities to create delicious, nutritious meals. From vegetable-based proteins like lentils and chickpeas to lean animal proteins such as chicken, fish, and turkey, the options are plentiful and can cater to various dietary preferences and requirements.

Incorporating high protein, low GI foods into your diet is a strategy that supports not only immediate blood sugar control and satiety but also long-term health goals. This balanced approach to eating promotes a sustainable, nutrient-rich diet that can enhance metabolic health, support weight management, and contribute to overall well-being. Whether you're managing diabetes, looking to lose weight, or simply aiming to eat healthier, the inclusion of high protein, low GI foods offers a solid foundation for achieving your dietary and health objectives.

Plant-Based Proteins and Low GI

Incorporating Plant Proteins for a Balanced Diet

The integration of plant-based proteins into a low glycemic index (GI) diet represents a holistic approach to nutrition that supports both metabolic health and environmental sustainability. Plant-based proteins, when combined with low GI foods, offer a powerful synergy that can enhance overall health, aid in weight management, and reduce the risk of chronic diseases. This section explores the benefits of plant-based proteins in the context of a low GI diet and offers guidance on how to incorporate these nutrients effectively.

Nutritional Benefits: Plant-based proteins come from sources that are naturally low in saturated fat and devoid of cholesterol, making them heart-healthy options. Many of these sources, such as legumes, lentils, chickpeas, and beans, are also low

GI foods, providing a double benefit of stable blood sugar levels and high-quality protein. In addition to protein, plant-based sources are rich in fiber, vitamins, minerals, and antioxidants, contributing to improved digestion, reduced inflammation, and enhanced nutrient intake.

Weight Management: The fiber content in plant-based proteins promotes satiety, helping to control appetite and reduce overall calorie intake. This can be particularly beneficial for weight loss or maintenance, as the combination of protein and fiber helps to keep you feeling full longer. Moreover, the low GI nature of these foods ensures a slow and steady release of energy, preventing blood sugar spikes and crashes that can lead to increased hunger and overeating.

Disease Prevention: Diets high in plant-based proteins and low GI foods are associated with a lower risk of developing chronic diseases such as type 2 diabetes, heart disease, and certain cancers. The low saturated fat content and absence of cholesterol in plant proteins contribute to heart health, while the low GI aspect supports stable blood sugar levels, reducing the risk of insulin resistance and diabetes.

Environmental Sustainability: Choosing plant-based proteins over animal sources can also have a positive impact on the environment. Plant-based diets require less water and land and generate lower greenhouse gas emissions compared to diets high in animal products. By incorporating more plant proteins into your diet, you're not only making a healthful choice but also contributing to a more sustainable food system.

Incorporating Plant-Based Proteins into Your Diet: To enjoy the benefits of plant-based proteins in a low GI diet, consider the following tips:
- Include a variety of plant proteins in your meals

to ensure a complete amino acid profile. Combine grains with legumes, for example, rice with beans or lentils with barley.

- Explore alternative protein sources such as tofu, tempeh, and edamame. These soy-based products are excellent low GI protein options that can be used in a wide range of dishes.

- Use nuts and seeds as a protein boost in salads, smoothies, or as snacks. Almonds, walnuts, chia seeds, and flaxseeds are not only rich in protein but also in healthy fats.

- Experiment with whole grains like quinoa and amaranth, which offer both protein and low GI carbohydrates.

Adopting a diet rich in plant-based proteins and low GI foods is a strategic approach to nutrition that supports long-term health and well-being. By making conscious dietary choices, individuals can enjoy the myriad benefits of these nutrients, from improved metabolic health and weight management to reduced disease risk and environmental impact.

Practical Applications

Creating a Low GI, High Protein Meal Plan

Planning Your Diet for Optimal Health

A diet that combines low glycemic index (GI) foods with high-quality protein sources is a powerful tool for maintaining stable blood sugar levels, supporting weight management, and promoting overall health. Creating a meal plan that incorporates these principles can help you achieve your health goals while enjoying delicious and nutritious meals. This section provides guidance on how to plan a low GI, high protein diet for optimal health.

Understanding Your Nutritional Needs: Before diving into meal planning, it's important to assess your individual nutritional needs, which can vary based on age, sex, weight, activity level, and health goals. Consider consulting with a healthcare provider or a registered dietitian to determine your specific protein and calorie requirements.

Building a Balanced Plate: A well-balanced meal includes sources of low GI carbohydrates, high-quality protein, healthy fats, and plenty of vegetables. Aim for half your plate to be filled with non-starchy vegetables, one quarter with low GI carbohydrates, and the remaining quarter with high protein foods.

Meal Planning Tips:

1. Start with Protein: Choose your protein sources for each meal first, focusing on lean meats, fish, dairy, and plant-based options like beans, lentils, and tofu. Then, build the rest of your meal around this protein source.

2. Incorporate Low GI Carbohydrates: Select low GI carbohydrates such as quinoa, sweet potatoes,

barley, and legumes. These foods will provide sustained energy without causing significant spikes in blood sugar levels.

3. Add Healthy Fats: Include sources of healthy fats like avocados, nuts, seeds, and olive oil to enhance flavor, increase satiety, and provide essential fatty acids.

4. Vary Your Vegetables: Fill at least half your plate with a variety of colorful vegetables. The more colors you include, the wider the range of nutrients you'll consume.

5. Plan Snacks Wisely: Opt for snacks that combine a low GI carbohydrate with a protein or healthy fat to keep you satisfied between meals. Examples include apple slices with almond butter or Greek yogurt with berries.

Sample Low GI, High Protein Meal Plan:

- Breakfast: Scrambled eggs with spinach, tomatoes, and whole grain toast.
- Lunch: Quinoa salad with grilled chicken, mixed greens, avocado, and a lemon-olive oil dressing.
- Dinner: Baked salmon with a side of steamed broccoli and sweet potato mash.
- Snacks: Greek yogurt with mixed berries; hummus with carrot and cucumber sticks.

Preparation Tips:

- Batch Cook: Prepare and cook your proteins and low GI grains or legumes in bulk to save time during the week.
- Use Fresh and Frozen Vegetables: Both fresh and frozen vegetables are nutritious. Keep a variety on hand for convenience.
- Experiment with Spices: Enhance the flavor of your meals with a variety of spices and herbs, which can make even the simplest meals feel

gourmet.

Creating a low GI, high protein meal plan is about finding a balance that works for your lifestyle and preferences. With some planning and creativity, you can enjoy a diverse range of meals that support your health goals and satisfy your taste buds. Remember, the key to a successful diet is not just about the foods you include but also about ensuring variety and balance to meet your nutritional needs.

Shopping and Preparing Low GI, High Protein Foods

Tips for Grocery Shopping and Meal Prep

Adopting a diet rich in low glycemic index (GI) and high-protein foods requires thoughtful grocery shopping and meal preparation strategies. These habits ensure you have the right ingredients on hand to create nutritious meals that align with your health goals. Here are practical tips to streamline your shopping and meal prep process, making it easier to enjoy a balanced and healthful diet.

Grocery Shopping Tips:

1. Make a List: Before heading to the grocery store, plan your meals for the week and make a detailed shopping list. This helps you stay focused, saves time, and reduces impulse buys that might not fit into your low GI, high-protein diet.

2. Shop the Perimeter: Most grocery stores are designed with fresh produce, meats, and dairy products around the perimeter. Start your shopping here to fill your cart with fresh, whole foods high in protein and low in GI.

3. Choose Whole Grains: Look for whole grain options like quinoa, barley, and rolled oats. These foods are lower in GI compared to their refined counterparts and provide additional fiber and nutrients.

4. Select Lean Proteins: Opt for lean cuts of meat, poultry, and fish. Plant-based proteins like beans, lentils, chickpeas, and tofu are also excellent choices that offer both low GI carbohydrates and high-quality protein.

5. Read Labels: For packaged foods, read nutrition labels carefully. Look for items with low added sugars and high fiber content, as these are

indicators of lower GI foods.

6. Buy in Bulk: Purchasing non-perishable items like whole grains, legumes, and nuts in bulk can save money in the long run. Store them properly to extend their shelf life.

Meal Prep Tips:

1. Batch Cook: Prepare large batches of low GI grains and legumes at the beginning of the week. Cooked quinoa, brown rice, or lentils can be refrigerated and used as a base for various meals throughout the week.

2. Prep Vegetables: Wash, chop, and store vegetables in the fridge for easy access. Having ready-to-eat veggies makes it simpler to include them in meals or grab them for a quick snack.

3. Protein Prep: Marinate and cook your protein

sources in advance. Grilled chicken, baked fish, and tofu can be refrigerated and added to salads, wraps, or stir-fries for quick, protein-packed meals.

4. Use Freezer-Friendly Meals: Prepare and freeze meals that reheat well, such as soups, stews, and casseroles. This is a great way to ensure you always have a healthy meal on hand, even on busy days.

5. Portion and Store: Divide cooked meals into single servings and store them in containers. This makes it easy to grab a balanced meal without having to cook from scratch every time.

6. Snack Preparation: Prepare healthy snacks in advance, such as portioning nuts and seeds, cutting up vegetables, or making a batch of hummus. Keeping these ready-to-eat snacks on hand can help prevent reaching for high GI alternatives.

By implementing these shopping and meal prep strategies, you can maintain a diet that supports your health without spending excessive time in the kitchen. Planning ahead and preparing ingredients or meals in advance are key steps to successfully eating a balanced diet of low GI, high-protein foods.

The Recipes

Low Glycemic, High Protein Recipes

Breakfasts to Start Your Day Right

Starting your day with a breakfast that's both low in glycemic index (GI) and high in protein can set the tone for balanced blood sugar levels and sustained energy throughout the morning. Here are six delicious recipes designed to do just that:

1. Quinoa & Berry Breakfast Bowl
- Ingredients: Cooked quinoa, mixed berries (strawberries, blueberries, raspberries), a dollop of Greek yogurt, a sprinkle of chia seeds, and a handful of crushed walnuts.
- Instructions: In a bowl, layer cooked quinoa with Greek yogurt and fresh berries. Top with chia seeds and walnuts for added protein and omega-3 fatty acids.

2. Spinach & Feta Omelette

- Ingredients: Eggs, fresh spinach, crumbled feta cheese, diced tomatoes, and herbs (such as dill or chives).

- Instructions: Whisk eggs and pour into a heated, non-stick skillet. Add spinach and tomatoes until slightly wilted. Sprinkle feta cheese and herbs on one half, fold over, and serve when the cheese is slightly melted.

3. Almond Butter & Banana Chia Pudding

- Ingredients: Chia seeds, unsweetened almond milk, almond butter, sliced banana, and a dash of cinnamon.

- Instructions: Mix chia seeds with almond milk and let sit overnight in the fridge. In the morning, stir in almond butter, top with banana slices, and sprinkle with cinnamon.

4. Cottage Cheese Pancakes

- Ingredients: Cottage cheese, eggs, oats, vanilla extract, and a touch of honey. Serve with fresh berries.

- Instructions: Blend cottage cheese, eggs, oats, vanilla, and honey until smooth. Cook spoonfuls in a non-stick skillet until golden brown. Serve with a berry compote for a low GI topping.

5. Avocado & Egg Toast on Sprouted Grain Bread

- Ingredients: Sliced avocado, poached or scrambled eggs, sprouted grain bread, and a sprinkle of chili flakes.
- Instructions: Toast sprouted grain bread, mash avocado on top, and add your cooked eggs. Season with chili flakes, salt, and pepper.

6. Greek Yogurt Smoothie with Spinach and Berries

- Ingredients: Greek yogurt, a handful of spinach, mixed berries, a tablespoon of flaxseed, and unsweetened almond milk.
- Instructions: Blend all ingredients until smooth.

Add a bit of water or ice to achieve your desired consistency. This smoothie packs protein, fiber, and essential nutrients to kickstart your day.

Each of these recipes is designed to provide a balanced combination of low GI carbohydrates and high-quality protein, ensuring you start your day on the right foot. Experiment with these options throughout the week to enjoy a variety of flavors and nutrients that support your health goals.

Energizing Lunches

Fuel your midday meal with these energizing, low glycemic, high protein lunch recipes. Perfect for keeping blood sugar levels stable and keeping you satiated throughout the afternoon.

1. Turkey and Quinoa Stuffed Peppers
- Ingredients: Bell peppers, ground turkey, cooked quinoa, diced tomatoes, onions, garlic, cumin, and shredded cheese.
- Instructions: Sauté onion and garlic, then brown the ground turkey with cumin. Mix in cooked quinoa and diced tomatoes. Cut bell peppers in half and remove seeds. Stuff the peppers with the turkey-quinoa mixture, top with cheese, and bake until peppers are tender.

2. Lentil Salad with Grilled Chicken
- Ingredients: Cooked lentils, grilled chicken breast (sliced), cherry tomatoes, cucumber, feta cheese,

olive oil, lemon juice, and herbs (parsley or mint).

- Instructions: Combine lentils, cherry tomatoes, and cucumber in a bowl. Top with slices of grilled chicken and crumbled feta cheese. Dress with olive oil, lemon juice, and fresh herbs before serving.

3. Chickpea and Avocado Wrap

- Ingredients: Whole grain wraps, mashed avocado, canned chickpeas (rinsed and drained), shredded carrots, baby spinach, and a squeeze of lime juice.

- Instructions: Spread mashed avocado onto whole grain wraps. Top with chickpeas, shredded carrots, and baby spinach. Drizzle lime juice over the filling before rolling up the wraps tightly.

4. Tofu and Vegetable Stir-Fry

- Ingredients: Firm tofu (cubed and pressed), assorted vegetables (broccoli, bell pepper, snap peas), soy sauce, ginger, garlic, and quinoa or brown rice for serving.

- Instructions: Stir-fry tofu until golden in a bit of oil. Remove and set aside. In the same pan, stir-fry vegetables with ginger and garlic. Add tofu back to the pan, splash with soy sauce, and stir until everything is heated through. Serve over cooked quinoa or brown rice.

5. Spinach and Feta Turkey Burgers

- Ingredients: Ground turkey, crumbled feta cheese, chopped spinach, minced garlic, onion powder, and whole grain buns.

- Instructions: In a bowl, mix ground turkey with feta cheese, chopped spinach, garlic, and onion powder. Form into patties and grill until fully cooked. Serve on whole grain buns with your choice of toppings like lettuce, tomato, and avocado.

6. Mediterranean Chickpea Salad

- Ingredients: Canned chickpeas (rinsed and

drained), diced cucumber, cherry tomatoes, red onion, kalamata olives, feta cheese, olive oil, lemon juice, and fresh herbs (such as parsley or oregano).

- Instructions: Combine chickpeas, cucumber, cherry tomatoes, red onion, and kalamata olives in a bowl. Add crumbled feta cheese. Dress the salad with olive oil, lemon juice, and a sprinkle of fresh herbs. Mix well and serve chilled.

7. Butternut Squash and Black Bean Bowl

- Ingredients: Roasted butternut squash cubes, black beans (rinsed and drained), quinoa, avocado slices, lime wedges, and a sprinkle of chili powder.
- Instructions: Serve roasted butternut squash and black beans over cooked quinoa. Add avocado slices on top and squeeze lime juice over the bowl. Sprinkle with chili powder for a touch of heat.

8. Grilled Salmon with Asparagus and Wild Rice

- Ingredients: Salmon fillets, fresh asparagus, wild rice, olive oil, lemon slices, and dill for seasoning.
- Instructions: Grill salmon fillets and asparagus spears until the salmon is flaky and asparagus is tender, seasoning both with olive oil and dill. Serve with cooked wild rice, garnishing with lemon slices for added flavor.

These eight recipes offer a variety of flavors and nutrients, ensuring your lunches are not only healthful but also delicious and satisfying. Incorporating these low glycemic, high protein meals into your weekly routine can help maintain energy levels, support weight management, and contribute to overall well-being. Experiment with these recipes and adjust ingredients according to your preferences to keep your lunches exciting and nutritious.

Satisfying Dinners

End your day on a high note with these satisfying, low glycemic, high protein dinner recipes. Each dish is designed to provide a balanced blend of nutrients to support your health goals, while also ensuring a delicious end to your day.

1. Zucchini Noodles with Lean Beef Meatballs
- Ingredients: Ground lean beef, grated Parmesan, minced garlic, chopped parsley, egg, zucchini (spiralized), and homemade tomato sauce.
- Instructions: Mix beef with Parmesan, garlic, parsley, and egg. Form into meatballs and bake until cooked through. Serve over spiralized zucchini noodles with homemade tomato sauce.

2. Cauliflower Rice Stir-Fry with Shrimp
- Ingredients: Cauliflower (riced), shrimp (peeled and deveined), mixed bell peppers, snap peas, onions, garlic, soy sauce (low sodium), and sesame

oil.

- Instructions: Sauté onions and garlic in sesame oil, add shrimp, and cook until pink. Add bell peppers and snap peas, stir-frying until just tender. Mix in riced cauliflower and soy sauce, cooking until heated through.

3. Baked Chicken with Mediterranean Vegetables

- Ingredients: Chicken breasts, zucchini, eggplant, bell peppers, cherry tomatoes, olives, olive oil, lemon juice, and mixed herbs (oregano, basil).
- Instructions: Toss vegetables with olive oil, lemon juice, and herbs. Place chicken breasts in a baking dish, surround with the vegetable mix, and bake until chicken is cooked and vegetables are tender.

4. Grilled Portobello Mushrooms with Quinoa Salad

- Ingredients: Large Portobello mushrooms,

cooked quinoa, arugula, cherry tomatoes, cucumber, feta cheese, balsamic vinegar, and olive oil.

- Instructions: Grill Portobello mushrooms until tender. Mix quinoa with arugula, cherry tomatoes, cucumber, and feta cheese. Dress the salad with balsamic vinegar and olive oil and serve with the grilled mushrooms.

5. Turkey Chili with Sweet Potato

- Ingredients: Ground turkey, diced sweet potatoes, canned tomatoes, black beans (rinsed and drained), onions, garlic, chili powder, cumin, and chicken broth.

- Instructions: Sauté onions and garlic until translucent. Add ground turkey, cooking until browned. Stir in sweet potatoes, tomatoes, black beans, chili powder, cumin, and chicken broth. Simmer until the sweet potatoes are tender. Serve hot with a dollop of Greek yogurt if desired.

6. Salmon and Asparagus Foil Packs

- Ingredients: Salmon fillets, asparagus spears, lemon slices, olive oil, dill, salt, and pepper.
- Instructions: Place each salmon fillet on a piece of foil. Top with asparagus, lemon slices, a drizzle of olive oil, and season with dill, salt, and pepper. Fold foil around the salmon and vegetables to seal. Grill or bake until salmon is cooked through and asparagus is tender.

7. Eggplant and Chickpea Curry

- Ingredients: Cubed eggplant, canned chickpeas (rinsed and drained), diced tomatoes, coconut milk, onion, garlic, ginger, curry powder, spinach, and cilantro for garnish.
- Instructions: Sauté onion, garlic, and ginger until softened. Add curry powder, stirring until fragrant. Add eggplant, chickpeas, tomatoes, and coconut milk, simmering until eggplant is tender. Stir in spinach until wilted. Garnish with cilantro and serve with a side of brown rice or quinoa.

8. Stuffed Bell Peppers with Ground Turkey and Quinoa

- Ingredients: Bell peppers, ground turkey, cooked quinoa, diced tomatoes, onions, garlic, shredded cheese (optional), and spices (cumin, paprika).
- Instructions: Sauté onions and garlic, add ground turkey and spices, cooking until browned. Mix in quinoa and diced tomatoes. Cut the tops off the bell peppers and remove the seeds. Stuff peppers with the turkey-quinoa mixture, top with cheese if using, and bake until the peppers are tender and filling is hot.

These eight satisfying dinner recipes offer a blend of low glycemic, high protein ingredients designed to support your health goals without sacrificing flavor. Whether you're cooking for one or preparing a meal for the family, these dishes are sure to please everyone at the table. Enjoy experimenting with these recipes, and feel free to adjust the ingredients to suit your dietary needs and preferences.

Snacks and Desserts

Healthy snacking and indulging in desserts can also align with your goals of maintaining a low glycemic, high protein diet. Here are six recipes that are not only nutritious but also satisfying for those mid-day cravings or after-dinner treats.

1. Greek Yogurt with Almond Butter and Cinnamon

- Ingredients: Plain Greek yogurt, almond butter, a sprinkle of cinnamon, and a few drops of vanilla extract.

- Instructions: Mix a dollop of almond butter into Greek yogurt. Add cinnamon and vanilla extract for flavor. This combination offers a creamy texture with a protein boost and a low GI.

2. Cottage Cheese and Pear Slices

- Ingredients: Low-fat cottage cheese and ripe pear slices.

- Instructions: Serve a bowl of cottage cheese with fresh pear slices on the side. The pear provides a sweet, low GI complement to the high-protein cottage cheese.

3. Avocado Chocolate Mousse
- Ingredients: Ripe avocados, cocoa powder, a sweetener of choice (such as stevia or monk fruit), vanilla extract, and a pinch of salt.
- Instructions: Blend ripe avocados with cocoa powder, sweetener, vanilla extract, and a pinch of salt until smooth. Chill before serving. This dessert offers a rich, creamy texture with the health benefits of avocado.

4. Protein-Packed Chia Seed Pudding
- Ingredients: Chia seeds, unsweetened almond milk, protein powder (vanilla or chocolate), and mixed berries for topping.
- Instructions: Mix chia seeds with almond milk and protein powder. Let the mixture sit until the

chia seeds have absorbed the liquid and the pudding has thickened. Top with mixed berries before serving.

5. Roasted Chickpeas with Spices

- Ingredients: Canned chickpeas (rinsed and drained), olive oil, and your choice of spices (such as paprika, garlic powder, cumin).
- Instructions: Toss chickpeas with olive oil and spices. Roast in the oven until crispy. This snack is perfect for a savory, crunchy treat that's high in protein and fiber.

6. Almond Flour Peanut Butter Cookies

- Ingredients: Almond flour, natural peanut butter, an egg, vanilla extract, and a sweetener of choice.
- Instructions: Mix all ingredients to form a dough. Roll into balls and press down with a fork on a baking sheet. Bake until golden. These cookies are low in GI due to almond flour and provide a good protein kick from the peanut butter.

These snack and dessert recipes combine the principles of low glycemic and high protein nutrition, ensuring you can enjoy tasty treats that support your health and wellness goals. Whether you need a quick snack or a satisfying dessert, these recipes offer delicious and healthful options to fit into your dietary plan.

Conclusion

The Path Forward: Integrating Low GI, High Protein Foods into Your Lifestyle

Embarking on a journey toward better health and wellness is a commendable goal, and the integration of low glycemic index (GI) and high protein foods into your diet is a powerful step in that direction. This approach not only supports stable blood sugar levels and sustained energy but also aids in weight management, improves metabolic health, and reduces the risk of chronic diseases. As you move forward, incorporating these nutritional principles into your lifestyle will become second nature, leading to lasting benefits for your health and well-being.

Adopting a Balanced Approach: Embracing a diet rich in low GI, high protein foods doesn't mean you have to sacrifice variety or enjoyment in your meals. It's about finding a balance that works for you, combining nutrient-dense foods with your personal preferences to create a diet that is both satisfying and health-promoting. Remember, the goal is to make sustainable changes that can be maintained over the long term, not to adhere to restrictive eating patterns that are difficult to follow.

Listening to Your Body: Each person's body responds differently to various foods and diets. Pay attention to how your body reacts to changes in your diet and adjust accordingly. If certain foods don't agree with you or don't satisfy you, explore other options that fit the low GI, high protein criteria. The key is to find a way of eating that feels good and is beneficial to your health.

Continuous Learning and Adaptation: Nutritional science is always evolving, and new research may offer additional insights into the benefits of low GI and high protein foods. Stay informed about the latest findings and be open to adjusting your dietary approach as new information becomes available. This proactive stance on learning will help you refine your diet to better suit your health needs and goals.

Seeking Professional Guidance: If you're unsure about how to start or if you have specific health concerns, consider consulting with a healthcare provider or a registered dietitian. These professionals can offer personalized advice and support to ensure your dietary choices align with your health objectives.

Building a Supportive Environment: Surround yourself with a community of like-minded individuals who share your commitment to healthy living. Whether it's family members, friends, or online communities, having support can make the journey more enjoyable and sustainable. Share recipes, tips, and experiences to learn from each other and stay motivated.

Integrating into Your Lifestyle: Ultimately, integrating low GI, high protein foods into your diet is about more than just what you eat; it's about creating a lifestyle that supports your overall health and happiness. Incorporate physical activity, stress management techniques, and adequate sleep into your routine to complement your dietary choices and enhance your well-being.

As you move forward on this path, remember that progress, not perfection, is the goal. Making small, consistent changes to your diet and lifestyle can lead to significant improvements in your health over time. Embrace the journey, celebrate your successes, and look forward to the positive impact that low GI, high protein foods can have on your life.

Appendices
Appendix A: Glycemic Index Chart of Common Foods

The Glycemic Index (GI) is a valuable tool for understanding how different foods can affect blood sugar levels. This chart provides the GI values for a variety of common foods, helping you make informed choices about what to include in your diet for better blood sugar management. Note that GI values can vary based on preparation methods and the ripeness of fruits and vegetables, so use this chart as a general guide.

Food Category	Food Item	Glycemic Index (Approx.)
Breads	Whole grain bread	55
	White bread	75
	Rye bread	65
Cereals	Rolled oats	55
	Instant oatmeal	70

Food Category	Food Item	Glycemic Index (Approx.)
	Corn flakes	80
Pasta/Noodles	Whole wheat pasta	55
	White pasta	45
	Rice noodles	50
Rice	Basmati rice	58
	Brown rice	50
	White rice	73
Legumes	Lentils	30
	Chickpeas	28
	Black beans	30
Vegetables	Carrots	39
	Broccoli	10
	Potatoes	78
Fruits	Apple	36
	Banana	51
	Watermelon	72
Dairy	Milk (full fat)	39
	Yogurt (low fat)	33
	Ice cream	61

Food Category	Food Item	Glycemic Index (Approx.)
Snacks	Chocolate	43
	Potato chips	56
	Popcorn	65

This glycemic index chart highlights the wide range of GI values across different food categories. Incorporating more low to medium GI foods into your meals can help maintain stable blood sugar levels, which is especially important for individuals managing diabetes, pre-diabetes, or looking to maintain a healthy weight. When planning your diet, consider pairing higher GI foods with sources of protein, healthy fats, and fiber to help balance the meal's overall glycemic impact.

Appendix B: Tips for Eating Out on a Low GI Diet

Eating out while adhering to a low glycemic index (GI) diet can seem challenging, but with the right strategies, you can enjoy dining experiences without compromising your health goals. Here are practical tips to help you navigate restaurant menus and make choices that align with a low GI lifestyle.

1. Research Restaurants in Advance:

- Look up menus online before visiting a restaurant. Many establishments provide nutritional information that can help you choose low GI options.

2. Start with a Salad:

- Begin your meal with a salad filled with non-starchy vegetables. Ask for the dressing on the side and opt for vinaigrettes or lemon juice to keep it low GI.

3. Choose Whole Grain or Sourdough Bread:

- If bread is part of your meal, request whole grain or sourdough options, which generally have a lower GI than white bread.

4. Select Lean Proteins:

- Opt for dishes that feature lean proteins such as chicken, fish, or legumes. These can help balance the meal's overall glycemic impact.

5. Ask for Substitutions:

- Don't hesitate to ask for substitutions that can lower the GI of your meal, such as replacing white rice or potatoes with quinoa, brown rice, or extra vegetables.

6. Be Mindful of Cooking Methods:

- Choose foods that are grilled, baked, steamed, or broiled rather than fried or breaded, as cooking methods can affect the GI of foods.

7. Control Portion Sizes:

- Restaurant portions can be generous. Consider sharing a dish or asking for half of your meal to be boxed up before you start eating to avoid overindulging.

8. Watch Out for Sugary Beverages:

- Stick to water, unsweetened tea, or coffee. Sugary drinks can significantly increase the GI of your meal.

9. Choose Low GI Sides:

- When selecting side dishes, opt for low GI options like mixed vegetables, salad, or legume-based dishes instead of fries or mashed potatoes.

10. Desserts:

- If you're craving something sweet, look for fruit-based desserts or those with dairy, like Greek yogurt with berries, which tend to have a lower GI than cakes or pastries.

Eating out on a low GI diet requires a bit of planning and awareness, but it doesn't have to limit your social life or enjoyment of food. By making informed choices and asking for modifications when needed, you can enjoy a wide range of dining experiences while staying true to your dietary goals.

Glossary of Terms

This glossary provides definitions for terms related to low glycemic index (GI) diets, high-protein foods, and general nutrition concepts mentioned throughout the guide. Understanding these terms can help you better navigate and implement the dietary strategies discussed.

1. Glycemic Index (GI): A numerical system that measures how much a carbohydrate-containing food increases blood glucose levels compared to pure glucose. Foods are ranked on a scale from 0 to 100, with higher values indicating a greater impact on blood sugar.

2. Glycemic Load (GL): A measure that takes into account both the glycemic index of a food and the amount of carbohydrate in a serving. It provides a more comprehensive view of how a food can affect blood sugar levels.

3. Carbohydrates: One of the three macronutrients found in food, carbohydrates are the body's primary source of energy. They are categorized into simple (sugars) and complex (starches and fibers) carbohydrates.

4. Protein: A macronutrient essential for building and repairing tissues, making enzymes and hormones, and supporting overall health. Proteins are made up of amino acids, some of which are essential and must be obtained from the diet.

5. Fats: A macronutrient important for energy, supporting cell growth, protecting organs, and helping with nutrient absorption. Fats can be saturated, unsaturated, or trans fats, with unsaturated fats considered the healthiest option.

6. Fiber: A type of carbohydrate that the body can't digest, found in plant-based foods. Fiber helps regulate the body's use of sugars, helping to keep hunger and blood sugar in check.

7. Insulin Resistance: A condition in which the body's cells do not respond properly to insulin, leading to higher blood sugar levels. Over time, it can lead to type 2 diabetes.

8. Whole Grains: Grains that contain all essential parts and naturally occurring nutrients of the entire grain seed. Examples include whole wheat, brown rice, oats, and quinoa.

9. Legumes: A class of vegetables that includes beans, peas, and lentils. They are high in protein, fiber, and various nutrients while being low in fat and glycemic index.

10. Macronutrients: The three main types of nutrients used by the body to provide energy: carbohydrates, proteins, and fats.

11. Amino Acids: Organic compounds that combine to form proteins. Amino acids are the building blocks of proteins and are essential for various bodily functions.

12. Metabolic Syndrome: A cluster of conditions that increase the risk of heart disease, stroke, and diabetes. It includes increased blood pressure, high blood sugar, excess body fat around the waist, and abnormal cholesterol levels.

13. Satiety: The feeling of being full and satisfied after eating, which can help control hunger and reduce overall calorie intake.

14. Antioxidants: Substances that can prevent or slow damage to cells caused by free radicals, thereby reducing inflammation and the risk of chronic diseases.

By familiarizing yourself with these terms, you

can gain a deeper understanding of the principles behind low GI and high-protein diets and how they contribute to health and wellness. This knowledge will empower you to make informed decisions about your diet and lifestyle.

Low Glycemic Foods, GI, and GL

This table of low glycemic (GI) foods along with their Glycemic Load (GL) can offer a practical guide for selecting foods that are beneficial for managing blood sugar levels and supporting a healthy diet. Below is a concise table featuring common low GI foods, their GI values, and their estimated GL per standard serving size. This table serves as a quick reference to help you make informed dietary choices.

Food Item	Quantity	GI	GL
Apple	1 medium (120g)	36	6
Pear	1 medium (120g)	38	4
Orange	1 medium (120g)	42	5
Berries	1 cup (120g)	25-40	3-6
Carrots, cooked	1 cup (200g)	39	2
Broccoli	1 cup chopped (91g)	10	1
Sweet Potato	1 medium (150g)	50	12
Lentils	1 cup cooked (200g)	30	5
Chickpeas	1 cup cooked (200g)	28	10

Food Item	Quantity	GI	GL
Black Beans	1 cup cooked (200g)	30	7
Quinoa	1 cup cooked (185g)	53	13
Rolled Oats	1 cup cooked (234g)	55	11
Barley	1 cup cooked (157g)	28	12
Whole Milk	1 cup (244g)	27	2
Yogurt, low-fat	1 cup (245g)	33	11
Almonds	1 oz (28g)	0	0
Hummus	1 tablespoon (15g)	6	0

Notes:

- The GI values are based on standardized testing and can vary due to factors like food preparation, ripeness, and specific varieties.

- The GL values provide a more accurate representation of how the food will impact blood sugar levels, considering both the GI and the amount of carbohydrate in the serving size.

- Low GI foods are classified as having a GI of 55 or less, medium GI foods have a GI of 56-69, and high GI foods have a GI of 70 or higher.

- A GL of 10 or less is considered low, indicating a

smaller impact on blood sugar levels, 11-19 is medium, and 20 or higher is considered high.

- This table aims to assist in dietary planning by highlighting the GI and GL of common foods, aiding in the selection of options that support stable blood sugar and overall health.

References and Further Reading

To deepen your understanding of low glycemic index (GI) and high-protein diets and their impact on health and wellness, the following references and resources are highly recommended. These materials offer valuable insights, detailed research findings, and practical advice to guide you in adopting a diet that supports stable blood sugar levels, weight management, and overall health.

Books:

1. "The Low GI Diet Revolution: The Definitive Science-Based Weight Loss Plan" by Dr. Jennie Brand-Miller. This book provides a comprehensive overview of the glycemic index, including how to choose low GI foods to manage weight and improve health.

2. "Protein Power: The High-Protein/Low Carbohydrate Way to Lose Weight, Feel Fit, and

Boost Your Health—in Just Weeks!" by Michael R. Eades and Mary Dan Eades. Explore the benefits of a high-protein diet and how it can help in weight loss and maintaining muscle mass.

3. "Good Carbs, Bad Carbs: An Indispensable Guide to Eating the Right Carbs for Losing Weight and Optimum Health" by Johanna Burani. Learn about the distinction between good (low GI) and bad (high GI) carbohydrates and their effects on your body.

Scientific Journals and Articles:
4. "Dietary glycemic index and glycemic load and the risk of type 2 diabetes: A systematic review and updated meta-analyses of prospective cohort studies" published in Nutrients. This article reviews the association between GI, glycemic load, and the risk of developing type 2 diabetes.

5. "Effects of high-protein diets on fat-free mass

and muscle protein synthesis following weight loss: a randomized controlled trial" published in The FASEB Journal. This study investigates the effects of high-protein diets on muscle mass during weight loss.

Websites:

6. The Glycemic Index Foundation (www.glycemicindex.com): An excellent resource for finding the GI values of various foods, understanding the glycemic index, and accessing low GI recipes.

7. The American Diabetes Association (www.diabetes.org): Offers resources and information on managing diabetes, including the importance of choosing low GI foods.

Online Courses and Videos:

8. Nutrition and Healthy Living course on Coursera or edX: Many universities offer free online courses that cover the basics of nutrition, including the roles of macronutrients and the glycemic index in health.

9. TED-Ed and YouTube: Search for videos on the glycemic index, high-protein diets, and their health benefits. These platforms feature content from nutrition experts and medical professionals.

By exploring these references and resources, you can gain a more nuanced understanding of how diet influences health and well-being. Whether you're looking for scientific research, practical diet plans, or educational videos, there's a wealth of information available to support your journey toward a healthier lifestyle.

Suggested Low Sugar Snacks & More:

You can purchase these items at your local health food store or easily order them from the comfort of your home via Amazon.

Keto low sugar Cacao
https://amzn.to/3OAMqlG

Hot Cocoa
https://amzn.to/3OylzG4

Low Glycemic snacks
https://amzn.to/3SBSgVr

More:

1. **Nuts:** Almonds, walnuts, and pistachios are excellent choices. They provide healthy fats, protein, and fiber. https://amzn.to/4bA2ga8

2. **Greek Yogurt:** Opt for plain Greek yogurt, which is high in protein and low in carbohydrates. https://amzn.to/3w8RHe2

3. **Vegetable Sticks with Hummus:** Carrot, celery, cucumber, and bell pepper sticks paired with hummus make a satisfying and low-glycemic snack. https://amzn.to/3SOyMOt

4. **Hard-Boiled Eggs:** Eggs are rich in protein and nutrients and have a minimal effect on blood sugar levels.

5. **Berries:** Strawberries, blueberries, and raspberries are delicious and low-glycemic fruits that can be enjoyed as a snack. https://amzn.to/3w4q9GA

6. **Cheese:** String cheese, cottage cheese, or slices of cheese are convenient and satisfying low-glycemic snacks. https://amzn.to/42z6NWe

7. **Avocado:** Avocado slices or guacamole are nutritious options packed with healthy fats and fiber. https://amzn.to/3wb0Z9r

8. Edamame: Steamed edamame pods are a tasty snack high in protein and fiber. https://amzn.to/42BaomJ

9. **Low-carb pancakes:** A delicious and satisfying option for individuals with diabetes, providing a tasty alternative to traditional pancakes while helping to better manage blood sugar levels and promote overall health. https://amzn.to/42xeaNS

These snacks can help keep blood sugar levels stable and provide sustained energy throughout the day.

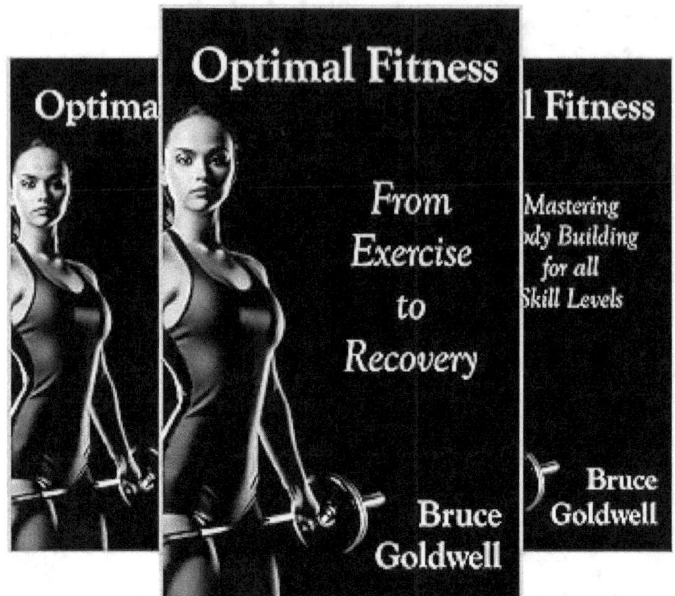

https://amzn.to/3uAQnzW

Optimal Fitness Series

"Discover the Secrets to a Longer, Healthier Life with this Comprehensive Collection of Lifestyle Transformation Books!

In this curated selection of empowering reads, you'll find a wealth of knowledge and guidance on how to rejuvenate your life and embrace a healthier, longer, and more vibrant future. These books offer a holistic approach to well-being, covering everything from nutrition and fitness to stress management and mental resilience.

Learn how to make mindful dietary choices that nourish your body, explore invigorating exercise routines, and tap into stress-reduction techniques that promote mental and emotional equilibrium. Dive into the science of longevity, uncovering the latest research on habits that can extend your lifespan while enhancing your quality of life.

Our collection of books is designed to inspire and motivate you to take proactive steps toward a healthier, more fulfilling existence. Whether you're embarking on a new wellness journey or seeking to refine your current lifestyle, these resources will empower you with the tools and knowledge needed to craft a brighter and longer future.

Join the countless individuals who have embraced these insights and made positive changes in their lives. Start your transformative journey today and embrace the potential for a life of vitality, happiness, and longevity."

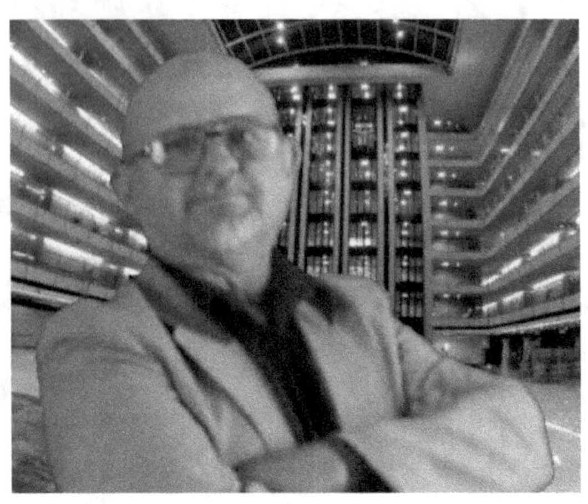

About The Author

Bruce Goldwell is a self-help/motivational author and creator of two captivating fantasy adventures, "Dragon Keepers" a six book series and "Starfighters Defending Earth" a three book series. He is an inspiring figure who has overcome significant challenges in his life. As a Vietnam veteran, he experienced homelessness for over ten years. During these difficult times, Bruce developed a compassionate heart and strong desire to uplift others. While living on the streets, he immersed himself in motivational literature at local bookstores, where he found solace in the works of renowned authors such as the creators of Chicken Soup for the Soul, Bob Proctor, and David Stanley, Elvis Presley's brother.

Inspired by the transformative impact of the film "The Secret," Goldwell penned his first book, "Mastery of Abundant Living: The Keys to Mastering the Law of Attraction." He had the honor of personally presenting the first autographed copy to Bob Proctor. Recognizing that young readers may not typically engage with self-help material, Goldwell brilliantly crafted a fantastical adventure series for teens. Within these enchanting stories, he weaves principles of success and powerful life lessons to ignite hope and encourage personal growth in younger audiences.

Driven by an unwavering belief in the power of his books to change lives, Bruce Goldwell's moving journey from homeless veteran to impactful author has resonated with thousands around the globe. His triumphant quest to help others is a testament to resilience, determination, and the transformative power of words.

Www.mykindlebooks.net